HERBAL MEDICINE & NATURAL REMEDIES FOR ALLERGIES

By Smith J. Offor

Table of Contents

INTRODUCTION

10 Homeopathic Treatments for Allergic Conditions

Your quality of life may be impacted by allergies, so it makes sense to be interested in any treatment that could lessen symptoms. However, if you're thinking about using a natural remedy, discuss it with your doctor first as some could come with serious side effects.

In the event of an allergic emergency, such as a life-threatening allergic reaction called anaphylaxis, no natural remedy is effective.

Exercise

Although the exact reason is unclear, regular exercise may be one of the most effective ways to help reduce allergic reactions, including respiratory allergies (related to breathing). Exercise has many health benefits and, of course, is not harmful to those with allergies when done in moderation.

The Benefits of Exercise

Allergy sufferers can exercise according to general population guidelines. In order to meet this requirement, you must engage in at least 75 minutes of vigorous exercise per week or 150 minutes of moderate exercise. These activities include strolling, jogging, cycling, using a treadmill, swimming, and more.

Side effects and cautions

If you have asthma or asthma that is aggravated by exercise, talk to your doctor about your exercise regimen. Observe any medical restrictions you may have. As your endurance increases, it's a good idea to gradually increase your exercise.

In addition, if you suffer from pollen allergies, check the pollen count before going outside.

Nasal irrigating

The term "nasal irrigation" can also refer to nasal rinse or saline lavage, and it is frequently used by allergy sufferers. It is a home remedy that involves flushing the nasal passages with sterile saltwater.

The Use of Irrigation

To relieve the signs of congestion, you can perform nasal irrigation every day, or even more than once. By buying a kit and following the directions, you can experiment with a nasal rinse.

Utilizing a neti pot and saline solution is one method. The solution drains from the other nostril after you pour it into one nostril from the pot. You can also use a bulb syringe or squeeze bottle.

When a patient is admitted to the hospital for an inpatient stay, a nasal rinse may occasionally be administered, especially for young children who are experiencing severe respiratory reactions.

RECIPE AND USES FOR NASAL OR SINUS RINSES

Advisory and negative effects

For nasal irrigation, only use distilled water or water that has been heated to a boil. Nasal irrigation using tainted tap water has caused amoeba infections in some cases. After every use, make sure to clean the device.

Before going to bed after nasal irrigation, it is best to wait at least an hour. That guarantees that all of the saline has been completely expelled from your sinuses and helps to stop coughing.

Supplement D

Anaphylaxis, allergic rhinitis (nasal congestion), allergic asthma, eczema, and vitamin D deficiency have all been linked to deficiencies in this vitamin. The release of chemicals that can cause allergy symptoms is regulated by this vitamin, which also plays a role in immune system cells.

The impact of acupuncture on allergic rhinitis was examined in a substantial systematic review that included several studies. The findings suggested that acupuncture may help allergy sufferers with their nasal symptoms, though the mechanism underlying this improvement was unclear. It was discovered that the procedure was risk-free and had no side effects.

Uses of Acupuncture

Along with traditional allergy treatment, acupuncture is frequently utilized as a complementary therapy. An acupuncturist would administer a series of weekly or biweekly treatments for a period of time, followed by any additional treatments that were required.

Side effects and cautions
Side effects are not typical with acupuncture, which is generally thought to be safe. Finding a practitioner who complies with your state's requirements for licensing, certification, or registration is preferable.

Treatment for allergies with acupuncture

Butterbur
Northern Asia, Europe, and some regions of North America are home to the shrub-like herb butterbur (Petasiteshybridus). The herb's extracts have been used in traditional medicine to treat asthma, allergic rhinitis, coughs, and migraine headaches as well as stomach cramps.

Uses for butterbur

Commercial butterbur extracts are created using the plant's leaves or roots. They can be purchased as tablets or capsules to be swallowed. Usually taken for a week or longer, the supplement is typically taken two to four times per day, especially during allergy season.

Side effects and warnings

Constipation, headaches, fatigue, nausea, vomiting, diarrhea, and sleepiness are a few of the potential butterbur side effects. Butterbur belongs to the ragweed plant family. Avoid butterbur and products that contain it if you have ragweed, marigold, daisy, or chrysanthemum allergies.

The raw butterbur herb should not be consumed alone, in tea, extract, or capsule form. It contains compounds called pyrrolizidine alkaloids, which can be toxic to the liver and lungs and may even cause cancer.

Any form of butterbur should not be consumed by children, pregnant or nursing women, people with kidney or liver disease, or children.

What Is A Butterbur?

Quercetin

As an antioxidant, quercetin aids in preventing cell deterioration. It lessens inflammatory proteins and cells, particularly in the skin. It is naturally present in foods like apples (with the skin on), berries, red grapes, red onions, capers, and black tea. It is also offered as a supplement.

Some people use it to treat allergic rhinitis, asthma, and atopic dermatitis (eczema).

Risks and negative effects

People with kidney disease, those who are pregnant or nursing, and those who are taking any medications should avoid taking quercetin.

Quercetin's health benefits.

Fatty acids with omega-3

It is crucial to consume omega-3 fatty acids.

You must obtain these fats from your diet since your body cannot produce them on its own.

Omega-3 fatty acids are found in foods like fish, walnuts, vegetable oil, flax seeds, and leafy greens.

Advisory and negative effects

Indigestion and a fishy aftertaste are possible side effects of fish oil. A minor "blood-thinning" effect of fish oil exists. Do not take fish oil without first talking to your doctor if you are taking coumadin (warfarin), heparin, or are at risk for bleeding issues. 20 Fish oil shouldn't be consumed two weeks prior to or following surgery.

Nettle that stings

The herb stinging nettle (Urticadioica) may lessen allergic rhinitis symptoms. Some people believe that this herbal supplement is one of the best for reducing allergy symptoms.

How to Use Stinging Nettle

You can drink stinging nettle tea. For the support of allergies, extracts can be found in a number of supplements.

Advisory and negative effects

Because stinging nettle has diuretic properties, it encourages your kidneys to produce more urine. It should not be used without first consulting a healthcare professional, especially if you are taking diuretics to treat fluid retention.

Recap

Although there hasn't been much research on this herb, stinging nettle, it may help with allergic rhinitis. Before taking it as a supplement, consult your doctor because it can increase urine production and act as a diuretic.

Utilizations for stinging nettle

- both prebiotics and probiotics.
- Live organisms, also known as "good" bacteria, or probiotics, help to strengthen the immune and digestive systems.
- Prebiotics are a type of fiber that promotes probiotic bacterial growth. They could enhance immune responses when added to infant formula.

The WAO also discovered that there is scant evidence in favor of using prebiotics.

Prebiotics may, however, be added as a supplement for infants who are not exclusively breastfed.

They point out that no research has been done on prebiotic supplements for expectant or nursing mothers.

As a result, they don't advocate using prebiotics during pregnancy.

What Prebiotics and Probiotics Are Used For

- Probiotics can be found in a range of products, such as kefir, yogurt, capsules, and supplemental drinks
- Fermented foods contain prebiotics
- Additionally, they come in tablet, capsule, and chewable form

Advisory and negative effects

In general, probiotics and prebiotics are secure.

However, if you are allergic to dairy products or any other potential ingredients, look for sources that are the safest for you.

Recap

Kefir, yogurt, and capsules are all sources of probiotics, or "good" bacteria.

Prebiotics are a type of fiber that encourages the development of probiotics. Both are regarded as being advantageous for immune health, but there isn't much information on whether they also help prevent allergies.

Allergy-Releasing Probiotics

- Oil from the seeds of black cumin
- Thymoquinone, one of the active chemical constituents in black cumin seed oil, has been linked to evidence of its potential to treat allergic rhinitis symptoms

What the Research Has Found

In one study, participants with allergic rhinitis were exposed to black cumin seed oil through the air or by rubbing it on their foreheads. They discovered that their episodes of sneezing, runny nose, and nasal itching had decreased.

To treat allergic rhinitis, a different study used nasal drops made from black cumin seed oil.

A six-week treatment program produced positive results in symptom relief.

How It Is Used

Both bulk and capsule forms of black cumin seed oil are offered for sale. Once or twice a day as a supplement is acceptable. Or, as in rhinitis studies, it can be rubbed on the skin, smelled, or used as drops in the nose.

Advisory and negative effects

Black seed oil doesn't appear to have any significant side effects, according to studies. On the other hand, when used topically, there is always a chance of a skin reaction. Before using it consistently, test a tiny amount on your skin. While using it for any length of time, keep an eye out for any reactions on your skin.

Safety of dietary supplements

The contents of a product may differ from what is stated on its label because supplements are not always tested for quality and are not heavily regulated. Safety for some people (e.g. g. nursing mothers, people taking medications, etc.) also hasn't been established.

Choose supplements that have been voluntarily submitted for testing by an impartial certifying body like U. S. ConsumerLab, NSF International, or the USP Pharmacopeia.

Brands that the U.S. S. Additionally, the Department of Agriculture (USDA) can lessen your risk of coming into contact with harmful chemicals and pesticides. Before taking a supplement for allergies or any other issue, always consult your healthcare professional.

6 natural remedies for allergic rhinitis
Describe allergic rhinitis

The nasal passages, sinuses, ears, and throat are all affected by the inflammatory condition known as allergic rhinitis. It happens when an allergic person inhales an allergen to which they are sensitive. It is also known as pollinosis and hay fever.

There are two varieties of allergic rhinitis. When exposed to airborne pollen and outdoor mold spores, those who suffer from seasonal allergies begin to experience symptoms in the spring, fall, or both seasons. Indoor allergens like house dust, pet dander, dust mites, and indoor molds cause perennial allergic rhinitis, a year-round condition.

Symptoms:

Itching, sneezing, runny nose, postnasal drip, as well as congestion in the nose, ears, and sinuses, are all signs of this allergy. During an allergy attack, there may also be fatigue and a general feeling of being "ill.". The severity of these symptoms varies from person to person.

Alternative Herbal Medicines for Allergies

Alternative treatments for allergic rhinitis may be available using herbal remedies.

These herbal remedies can not only lessen allergic symptoms, but also prevent them altogether if used wisely. Additionally, they can strengthen your body's tissues and organs, which will enhance your general health. The best herbs for treating allergies and other respiratory conditions are listed below.

Urticadioica, also called stinging nettle

Those unfortunate enough to unintentionally brush against its leaves are familiar with this plant. For many would-be gardeners, coming into contact with stinging nettles is painful, but it's also one of the best herbal remedies for allergic rhinitis. It can lessen inflammation caused by allergies without causing any of the side effects associated with using pharmaceuticals because it is an antioxidant, astringent, antimicrobial, and analgesic.

The spring season offers fresh nettle

The stinging properties of the leaves can be eliminated by cooking them, and like most other green leafy vegetables, you can add them to salads, soups, or stews. You can also make nettle tea using it once it has been dried.

Perillafrutescens, a perilla

A member of the mint family, this somewhat obscure herb can aid you in the fight against the signs and symptoms of allergic rhinitis. Numerous studies have demonstrated the value of perilla in the treatment of sinusitis, allergic asthma, allergic rhinitis, and eye irritation (another issue that many allergy sufferers face). It can also treat skin conditions brought on by allergies. It's important to point out that the perilla's essential oils have antidepressant properties and raise serotonin levels in the brain. In other words, in addition to lowering body inflammation, this miraculous herb also lifts your spirits and makes you feel better overall.

Hippocaerhamnoides, also known as sea buckthorn

With its thorny, grey twigs and bright orange, ovoid fruit, this plant quickly develops into a shrub or small tree. More than 190 nutrients and phytonutrients are found in sea buckthorn. This extraordinarily nutrient-rich berry provides a wide range of organic acids, tannins, quercetin, provitamin A, vitamin E, a substantial amount of vitamin C, and B complex vitamins. In addition, it is rich in superoxide dismutase (SOD), an enzyme that is essential for maintaining respiratory health. People with allergic rhinitis, asthma, chronic coughs, and other breathing problems benefit greatly from sea buckthorn. Its special nutrient composition enhances the condition of the mucous membranes, mouth, and eyes. There are many sea buckthorn products available on the market right now, but you should choose wisely and only purchase from a reputable business that has high standards for quality.

Petasiteshybridus is the butterbur

In marshes in North America, Europe, and Asia, the butterbur shrub can be found. It has historically been used to treat conditions like pain, headaches, fevers, and digestive issues. In more recent years, it has also been used to treat hay fever, migraines, uti, and headaches in general, including migrainous headaches. Butterbur has also been the subject of scientific investigation, with encouraging outcomes. According to one such study, this herb functions similarly to the over-the-counter allergy drug Zyrtex. Extracts from the root, rhizome, or leaves are used in butterbur products. Since this herb contains some alkaloids (PAs) that are harmful to humans, you shouldn't use it in its raw form. Always choose items with the phrase "PA-free" on the label.

Ginger is called Zingiberofficinale

Ginger is a herb that is safe and very powerful. The fact that it calms the digestive system and enhances circulation makes it very advantageous to your overall health in addition to its culinary uses. Ginger functions as a powerful antiviral, natural antihistamine, and immune builder. Try drinking some ginger tea to relieve headaches and sinus congestion. Inhale the steam from your tea as you continue to sip. Both fresh and dried ginger are available commercially. Additionally, you can combine it with other herbs, like the potent natural healer turmeric.

Achilleamillefolium, also known as yarrow

Native to the British Isles, yarrow is a perennial herb that is also widely used in Asia and Europe. This versatile herb has antiseptic, stomachic, antispasmodic, astringent, and diaphoretic properties. Yarrow has a long history of use for the treatment of fevers, the flu, and colds. It is also an effective treatment for allergic rhinitis. The respiratory system benefits greatly from this herb's anti-microbial and anti-catarrhal properties, and it also treats sinusitis and dust allergies. Yarrow is available as a tincture or in the form of tea. This herb has a strong flavor, so it should only be used internally daily for two weeks in a row. In addition, since ragweed and this herb are related, you should stay away from it if you have ragweed allergies.

Effective Medicine Can Be Made from Natural Plants

The signs of allergic rhinitis and other respiratory conditions can be relieved with herbal treatments. They can also strengthen your immune system and delay the onset of an allergic reaction if used wisely and proactively. But you must speak with a specialist before attempting any new treatment.

HOME REMEDIES FOR ALLERGY RELIEF

Allergies: What Are They?

An exaggerated or pathological immunological reaction (such as by sneezing, difficult breathing, itching, or skin rashes) to substances, situations, or physical states is what is referred to as an allergy.

In other words, allergies result from immune system hypersensitivity, which triggers negative reactions that can have a negative impact on the entire body.

The most frequent triggers of allergies include things like dust, certain foods, animal fur, outdoor pollen, and dust.

When your body reacts to allergens, histamine is produced.

Histamine functions by helping to neutralize the allergen, which causes allergy symptoms to appear.

Immunoglobulin E (IgE) antibodies, which are produced by the immune system and lead to widespread symptoms, are what cause allergic reactions.

Allergies can be divided into a number of broad categories, including:

Seasonal allergies, also known as rhinitis or hay fever, typically get worse when pollen levels rise or change, like in the spring or fall.

- seasonal allergies that are persistent
- allergies to certain foods, like shellfish

- allergies to drugs or medications
- indoor allergies, such as those caused by mold or dust
- eye or skin allergies
- allergies to pets or animals, including those to dogs, cats, insects, etc
- Anaphylaxis is a severe, potentially fatal allergic reaction that can occur in response to numerous allergens

Symptoms/Causes

The symptoms brought on by allergies differ from person to person, depend on the trigger, and change according to how severe the allergy is. The following are examples of typical allergy symptoms:

- Runny nose, itchy nose, congestion, and stuffiness

- Skin rash, redness, hives, dryness, peeling or itchiness
- mouth and lips that tingle or itch
- swelling of the face, throat, lip, or tongue
- vomiting and nauseousness
- stomach cramps and diarrhea
- Symptoms of asthma, such as coughing, wheezing, and breathing difficulties can occasionally be brought on by allergies
- dizziness, lightheadedness, and in extreme cases, unconsciousness

How Do Allergies Develop?

It can be challenging to identify the specific allergens that are causing your symptoms because there are so many different types of allergies. The following are some of the most typical causes of allergies.

- pollen from grass, trees, and other plants.
- Dust, such as the varieties that surround your home.
- Certain foods, particularly those known to be the most common triggers of food allergies, such as gluten, dairy, tree nuts (especially peanuts), eggs, soy, and shellfish.
- stings and bites from insects.
- Pet hair and dander.

Mold

- certain drugs, including antibiotics.

- Latex, such as the kind used to make condoms or latex gloves.

- Personal care and cosmetics with added fragrances (the root of so-called "fragrance sensitivities").

- Smoking, including cannabis, which is associated with asthma in some cases.

- Conventional Treatments for Allergies.

The following approaches are frequently used to treat allergies:

- Decongestants available over-the-counter
- Antihistamines are medications that stop the chemicals that trigger allergic reactions from releasing into the body
- Immunotherapy medications
- droplets for the eyes
- creams for the skin, such as those containing steroids or antihistamines
- Inflammation is managed with corticosteroids
- Elimination diets to treat food allergies, such as dairy- and gluten-free diets

In case of an attack, someone with severe allergies may also carry an emergency epinephrine auto-injector (Epipen).

Some experts feel that the conventional treatment approaches above (besides an elimination diet) are not the best ways to manage allergies because they don't fix the underlying causes.

When it comes to allergies, what's important to understand is that when your immune system produces an allergic reaction to something it's because it senses that something is not right within your body. For true allergy relief, you need to find the underlying cause and strengthen your natural defense system rather than just treating the symptoms of allergies (such as itchy skin or watery eyes, for example).

When we take prescribed medications or over-the-counter products for allergies, these can disturb natural processes of your immune system and have other deleterious effects like altering our pH balance. To keep symptoms at bay, you will always have to take a drug because your body doesn't learn how to adapt to allergens.

Drugs, drops, creams, and other allergy-related items can reduce and mask symptoms, but they don't deal with the underlying issue.

Natural Allergy Relief Options

What helps relieve allergies fast? Watching what you eat, getting plenty of fresh air and drinking enough water are some of the natural remedies that can relieve allergies by improving functions of the immune system.

It may take several weeks for your symptoms to subside, but they are likely to be better kept under control when you tackle the root causes. Here are nine ways to get natural allergy relief.

1. Eat an Anti-Inflammatory, Alkaline Diet

First and foremost, start eating an anti-inflammatory diet to reduce your risk for allergies and many other health problems.

Caring for your body with nutrient-dense foods gives your immune system the ability to repair itself, bringing it back into balance so it can fight off common allergies in your environment.

Here are some of the best foods and ingredients to incorporate into your diet to help you beat allergies:.

Garlic —What's so fantastic about garlic? Garlic is a natural antibiotic that helps ward off infections, viruses and even allergies. Eating or juicing two raw cloves of this powerful antioxidant may literally keep the doctor away. Some people choose to take garlic supplements because they don't want to smell like garlic, but the supplements do not work as well as the real herb does, so don't be deceived by this. Raw garlic eaten every day helps fight off all types of allergies because it boosts your immune system immensely.

Lemons —As most of us know, an alkaline body means better balance and immune function. Lemons and limes are excellent immune-boosting fruits and used for various afflictions, including allergies. Vitamin C and antioxidants that support the immune system are abundant in both of these fruits. Drinking lemon water throughout the day detoxifies the body and rids it of impurities. Mix the juice of one or two lemons or limes with olive oil to make a wonderful-tasting dressing for salads and veggie sandwiches.

Green leafy vegetables — Leafy greens (including spinach, kale, collard greens, romaine, arugula and watercress) are great sources of essential vitamins, minerals, antioxidants and enzymes that aid detoxification and help reduce inflammation.

Probiotic-rich foods — Probiotic foods support immune health and can help repair a damaged intestinal lining. Kefir, sauerkraut, kimchi, natto, yogurt, raw cheese, miso, and kombucha are some examples.

Bone broth — Bone broth, made from beef and chicken stock, is rich in many minerals and amino acids that support the treatment of leaky gut, thereby helping strengthen the immune system.

Coconut milk —The best alternative for cow's milk is coconut milk, which is free of dairy, lactose, soy, nuts and grains.

Almond butter and seeds —For people allergic to peanuts and peanut butter, almond butter is a safe and healthy alternative that provides healthy unsaturated fatty acids, fiber, minerals like riboflavin and magnesium, and even some antioxidants. Flaxseeds, chia seeds, pumpkin seeds and sunflower seeds are also great sources of healthy fats and fiber.

Gluten-free flours/grains — Instead of using wheat flour when you cook or bake, try coconut flour, almond flour, spelt flour, oat flour and rice flour, which are all gluten-free.

Breast milk — Studies shows that exclusive breastfeeding seems to have a preventive effect on the early development of asthma and atopic dermatitis.

Although it's not abundant in many foods, vitamin D is also important for immune function and may help manage allergy symptoms. In fact, certain studies have shown that children who live farther from the equator are more likely to develop allergies and suffer higher rates of hospital admissions due to allergic reactions.

You can get enough vitamin D by spending about 15 minutes in the sun most days without sunscreen and by eating foods like whole milk and some mushrooms for natural allergy relief.

2. Local Raw Honey (Bee Pollen)

Considering how good it tastes, having some raw honey every day to help control seasonal allergies may sound too easy to actually work well, but don't discount this ancient remedy. Taking a tablespoon of local, raw honey every day helps your body build a tolerance to the local pollen that is running amuck on your sinuses.

Researchers involved According to another study published in the Journal of Allergy, discovered that patients taking honey "reported a 60 percent lower total symptom score, twice as many asymptomatic days, and 70 percent fewer days with severe symptoms. They also used 50 percent less antihistamines compared to the control group that took conventional meds.

Try taking one tablespoon of raw local honey daily, such as by stirring some into tea, adding some to oatmeal along with cinnamon, or putting some in your smoothies.

What makes raw honey so powerful at reducing allergies? One reason is because it contains bee pollen, which is known to ward off infections and allergies and boost immunity.

The bees living in your area go from flower to flower collecting pollen that you are suffering from. It would make sense then that eating local raw honey will help build up your immunity to local pollen.

Honey also contains many enzymes that supports overall immune function, which helps with allergy relief.

3. Apple Cider Vinegar (ACV)

You can now find high-quality apple cider vinegar in most supermarkets, which is great considering it can help break up mucus and support lymphatic drainage.

Drinking a glass of water with a teaspoon of ACV and some fresh lemon juice is one of the best ways to wake up every morning. At the first sign of an allergy attack, put one teaspoon of ACV in your neti pot solution for a natural "sinus flush.

4. Quercetin

Quercetin is a polyphenol antioxidant that is naturally found in plant foods, such as cruciferous vegetables (like broccoli or cauliflower), onions/shallots, green tea and citrus fruits. Considered a bioflavonoid that stabilizes the release of histamines, it helps naturally control allergy symptoms.

The results of a 2020 study suggest that Quercetin possesses antiallergic properties that are known to inhibit histamine synthesis and proinflammatory mediators. Quercetin helps to reduce congestion by calming the airways' hyperactivity.

It is so powerful that researchers have found evidence suggesting that quercetin can help control peanut allergies, the leading cause of life-threatening/fatal allergy attacks. Various sources suggest that it is best to use quercetin as a long-term remedy, since it can take several months of use to start working.

People prone to seasonal allergies should start to take it a few weeks before spring arrives when trees and plants start to bloom.

5. Neti Pot

What is the best allergy relief for a runny nose? Neti pots are a natural remedy for allergies and many respiratory conditions because they help clear the sinuses and remove congestion.

Use of neti pots has been shown to help improve quality of life in sufferers of respiratory illnesses and cause little to no side effects.

Clearing the nasal passages of allergens and irritants, this form of "sinus irrigation" originated in the Ayurvedic medicine tradition hundreds of years ago. People living in India have been receiving astounding results from using neti pots for centuries, and now you can, too.

In order to achieve the highest level of sterility when using a neti pot, make sure the water is distilled. Using tap water can actually make your sinuses worse because it contains high levels of fluoride and chlorine.

If you don't want to use a neti pot, you could also try a salt water sinus rinse, which involves combining sea salt and warm water and inhaling it through one nostril.

6. Nettle that stings

A growing number of doctors are advising taking a freeze-dried preparation prior to the start of the hay fever season because studies have specifically shown that stinging nettle leaf naturally regulates histamines. It can also be taken as a tincture or as tea.

Other herbal treatments, according to specialists in sinus allergies, may help control symptoms by boosting the immune system and easing congestion.

- Ginger
- Turmeric.
- Yarrow.
- Shiitake mushrooms.
- Astralagus.
- Perillafrutescens, the perilla plant.
- Hippocaerhamnoides, also known as sea buckthorn.
- Butterbur, or Pctasitcshybridus.
- "Horehound" (Marrubiumvulgare)

7.Frankincense oil and eucalyptus oil

A fascinating study looked at the effectiveness of different essential oils in eliminating the highly allergic house mites and discovered that eucalyptus oil was among some of the most potent. The way that essential oils for allergies work is by reducing inflammation and enhancing the body's ability to rid itself of toxins, parasites, parasitic bacteria, and other harmful organisms that can cause attacks.

There are several ways to apply eucalyptus oil for seasonal allergy relief:

You can use eucalyptus oil as an antimicrobial agent in your laundry detergent, add a few drops to your neti pot, or breathe it in through a diffuser.

Add 25 drops of eucalyptus oil to each wash load during allergy season, especially if you or the kids are outside playing.

This eco-friendly, biodegradable addition to your natural detergents will help you stay allergy-free.

If your allergy symptoms are severe, combine eucalyptus oil and coconut oil, massage it into your chest and behind your ears, and diffuse the mixture throughout the day and at night.

Frankincense oil is another potent essential oil for controlling allergies. For years, Indian frankincense has been well-documented in scientific literature for its almost unbelievable ability to kill cancer, but its ability to prolong life doesn't stop there.

In a study reported in Phytotherapy Research, it was found that mice receiving 1–10 milligrams of frankincense orally experienced stimulation of their immune systems on multiple levels, including IgG,

IgM, and interferon. This indicates that frankincense has extremely potent effects on boosting the immune system.

Simply rub frankincense behind your ears and on your chest several times each day to incorporate it into your natural health regimen, or diffuse frankincense essential oil for about three hours each day in your home and office.

8. Probiotics

A healthy gut is the foundation of a powerful immune system, which is now widely recognized. The gastrointestinal (GI) tract houses more than 80% of your immune system's storage capacity. Research linking probiotic supplement use to a lower risk of allergies should not come as a surprise.

Probiotics are helpful "good bacteria" that reside in your GI tract and aid in protecting you from illnesses like allergies, infections, and viruses, among other things. They are being used more frequently to treat gut dysbiosis, which is an imbalance of bacteria in the microbiome, which in turn affects allergic diseases.

They are so effective that a study in the journal Pediatrics found that pregnant women who regularly take probiotics significantly lower the likelihood that their unborn children will develop allergies.

I strongly advise consuming probiotic supplements or probiotic foods, which can be made from ingredients found in your own backyard garden or sold at farmers markets, to obtain soil-based organisms.

9. To get rid of irritants, clean up your house.

To reduce your exposure to irritants and triggers like dust, fragrances, etc., there are many things you can do. Here are a few of the best adjustments you can make to your daily beauty, cleaning, and home maintenance routines to naturally relieve allergy symptoms:

- Take care not to wear perfume or burn scented candles in your house.
- Use hypoallergenic cosmetics, such as lotions, shampoos, and other items.

- Use hypoallergenic (or detergent without dyes or fragrances) laundry detergent. Avoid using softeners and dryer sheets

- For indoor air purification, use a humidifier. A high-efficiency particulate air (HEPA) filter might also be useful

- To keep your home dust-free, vacuum frequently, and wash linens, towels, and blankets frequently

- Keep windows closed during seasons of the year when outdoor allergens are prevalent

Be mindful of how your allergies may be impacted by houseplants and animals.

Risks and negative effects.

While the majority of the aforementioned supplements and advice can safely reduce allergic reactions, there are a few things to watch out for.

The majority of the time, mild to moderate allergies are not life-threatening and eventually go away. However, severe allergic reactions can be harmful and need to be treated by a doctor.

Severe allergic reactions, also known as anaphylaxis, can be brought on by contact with substances such as foods, medications, or insect stings. The following are examples of symptoms that typically impact the heart, blood vessels, or lungs:

- breathing difficulties
- chest constriction

- pain in the chest
- The blood pressure varies
- dizziness.
- fainting
- rash
- vomiting

Visit your doctor or the emergency room as soon as possible if you or your child exhibits these symptoms to avoid further issues.

If you have severe allergies, your doctor may recommend allergy shots or prescription asthma medications like bronchodilators and inhaled corticosteroids.

With your healthcare provider, go over these options, and think about trying the natural allergy relief methods mentioned above in addition to using medications.

Get Rid of Allergies Naturally

- herbs as supplements
- These can be consumed as a capsule, as drops, or as tea

According to allergist Tim Mainardi, MD, of New York City, you may already have one effective remedy for allergies in your kitchen. "Green tea is an effective natural antihistamin that is potent enough to actually affect allergy skin testing," he says.

To prevent congestion, consume two cups per day beginning about two weeks before the start of allergy season.

Both over-the-counter antihistamines and the herb butterbur, according to Mainardi, may prevent allergies. Another excellent option, in his opinion, is licorice root because it "raises your body's level of naturally produced steroids.". More research is required to confirm this, but it may also aid in releasing mucus, making it easier to breathe and suppressing coughing.

Before attempting herbal treatments, consult your doctor.

Some butterbur products contain a component that can harm your lungs and liver. A reaction to butterbur may also occur if you have an allergy to ragweed, marigolds, or daisies.

Licorice should also be used responsibly.

Large doses can result in heart issues and high blood pressure. Licorice supplements ought to be avoided by expectant mothers. They might result in premature labor.

Food Changes
According to Kathryn Boling, MD, a family medicine specialist at Mercy Medical Center in Baltimore, hot, spicy foods have an effect that can help clear nasal passages, which explains why your nose may start to run after finishing a plate of hot wings.

If you want to spice up your food, try adding cayenne pepper, spicy ginger, or the European and Asian plant fenugreek. Even though they aren't as hot, onions and garlic can still soothe a runny nose and relieve head congestion.

Check with your doctor to see if eliminating certain foods from your diet will also help with allergy symptoms. Dried fruits and some dairy products, such as some cheeses, can enlarge the blood vessels in your nose and exacerbate congestion.

In addition, Boling advises against eating melon, bananas, cucumbers, sunflower seeds, and chamomile for those who are allergic to ragweed, pollen, or other weed pollens. "These foods can all aggravate symptoms.

Make a list of the foods you believe might be triggering your allergies. Visit your doctor soon and bring this "food diary" with you.

Acupuncture

Sneezing, runny nose, puffy eyes, and other allergy symptoms have all been treated with this traditional Chinese technique.

A skilled practitioner will carefully insert hair-thin needles under your skin at various locations on your body during a session.

Dr. Thomas Burgoon, president of the American Academy of Medical Acupuncture, states that it is typical to see improvement even after the first treatment. For a period of six weeks, you might need two sessions if you have ongoing (chronic) allergies.

Nasal rinsing

To remove dust and pollen from your nose, use a Neti pot. One is available at the pharmacy down the street. This device has an extended spout that resembles a small teapot.

One nostril at a time, rinse with distilled or sterile water. To reduce allergy symptoms, do this twice daily, advises Mainardi.

Allergy-Proofing

Eliminating sneezing-inducing items from your home is the simplest way to prevent an allergy attack.

Remove allergens from rugs and furniture by vacuuming at least once a week. Whenever possible, use a HEPA filter.

What are the top all-natural treatments for allergies?

There are two main methods you can use to treat allergies naturally:

Adapt your environment and lifestyle to avoid allergens.

To lessen the symptoms when they appear, alter your diet or take a supplement.

preventing allergens

Knowing what you're allergic to will help you avoid these triggers by modifying your environment and daily routine. You can: to treat seasonal pollen allergies.

- Like you would check the weather, check the pollen count in your area.

- On days with a lot of pollen, stay indoors.
- When you're outside, think about wearing a mask.
- To keep pollen from entering your home, close your windows.
- A high-efficiency particulate air purifier (HEPA air purifier) might be used to purify the air in your house.

Try a saline rinse to clear your nose if you've been outside and are experiencing worsening allergy symptoms. This can assist in removing pollen that has built up in your nasal passages and may be the cause of your allergies.

Cleaning your home can help with allergy symptoms if you are also allergic to indoor triggers like dust or pet dander. Here are some recommendations you can use:

Dust mites can be removed from bedding by washing it in hot water and drying it on high at least twice a week.

Try using mattress covers and pillowcases that are dust mite-proof.

Try to vacuum your carpet or area rugs at least once every two weeks if you have them in your home.

Clean your bathroom to remove any mold or mildew that is readily apparent.

Try to keep your pet away from the furniture and from your bedroom to prevent pet allergies. Please be aware that your pet may bring indoor pollen with them from the outside.

Control of allergy symptoms

- Avoiding allergy triggers or anticipating a flare-up of your symptoms is not always possible

- Other herbal treatments can therefore aid in symptom reduction

- To stay hydrated in the spring and summer when it's warmer outside is one of the simplest advices

- This can lessen the discomfort and thickening of your mucus, which can help with allergy symptoms

There are additional supplements you can try to ease the effects of your allergies:.

Many foods contain quercetin, which is also available as a supplement. According to some studies, it might benefit allergies. Although quercetin is generally regarded as safe, it can interact with some medications and exacerbate any kidney issues that already exist.

You can either consume or supplement with stinging nettle. Small studies suggest it might help with allergies, but more research is required. Although it rarely does, stinging nettle can have minor side effects like nausea and vomiting.

You can take vitamin C supplements or find it in many foods. It might help with allergies, according to small studies. While vitamin C is generally regarded as safe, it can interact with some medications and have undesirable side effects, including flushing, headaches, and vomiting. At higher doses, this is especially true.

The butterbur shrub is where butterbur extract is found. Studies suggest that butterbur extract, which functions similarly to fexofenadine (Allegra) and cetirizine (Zyrtec), may be a useful allergy treatment. However, there are security worries that butterbur could cause cancer and liver damage. Butterbur-containing products shouldn't be consumed by expectant mothers.

What foods relieve allergy symptoms?

No specific food has been shown to be effective in treating allergies. The nutrients and substances found in many fruits, vegetables, and other foods, such as quercetin and vitamin C, may help with allergies.

Quercetin can be found in the following foods:

- asparagus, kale, onions, spinach, and broccoli are some examples of vegetables
- Fruits like blueberries, cherries, cranberries, and apples
- herbs, such as dill, oregano, and chives
- spices, including hot peppers
- beverages: such as red wine and black tea

The following list of foods contains vitamin C.

- vegetables, including cauliflower, red peppers, broccoli, Brussels sprouts, and cabbage.
- fruits, including kiwis, oranges, grapefruit, strawberries, and grapes.

It's important to be aware that grapefruit can cause a number of medications to interact before making dietary changes. Additionally, you might need to change the dosage of your blood thinner, warfarin (Coumadin), if you start consuming more leafy green vegetables.

Can honey treat allergies?

Perhaps you've heard that honey is good for allergies. Flowers and other plants that produce pollen are used by bees to make honey. Accordingly, the theory is that consuming local honey also exposes you to a small amount of local pollen, which will gradually reduce your susceptibility to seasonal allergies. Actually, allergy shots, a tried-and-true remedy for seasonal allergies, work on the same principle. .

Unfortunately, even when purchasing local honey from the same supplier, the quantity and type of pollen you receive can vary between batches. Although studies have not shown that honey helps to treat allergies, it can be a delectable addition to your diet. It's also crucial to be aware that babies younger than 12 months old shouldn't be given honey.

Why are natural allergy treatments advantageous?

Benefits of various natural remedies vary. If you consume a lot of quercetin and vitamin C, for example, it is likely that you also consume a lot of fruits and vegetables. This implies that your diet is probably going to have a lot of other nutritional advantages.

One of the main advantages of using other natural remedies, such as dietary changes and supplements, is avoiding the potential side effects of using over-the-counter medications.

What negative effects can OTC allergy medications have?

The majority of over-the-counter allergy medications have been in use for a very long time, and they are typically safe and well tolerated. Although some people might prefer to avoid them, these medications can still have side effects. The various adverse effects of typical over-the-counter allergy medications are listed below.

Antihistamines

Some of the most widely used and recognized allergy medications are oral antihistamines. Antihistamines frequently cause the following side effects.

Drowsiness

- the mouth is dry.
- Urinating is difficult.

With more recent antihistamines like fexofenadine (Allegra) or cetirizine (Zyrtec), these side effects are typically much milder; however, with older antihistamines like diphenhydramine (Benadryl), they are typically worse.

People over 65 years old may also experience them more severely.

nostril spray

There are numerous types of nasal sprays for allergies that contain various medications, including steroids, decongestants, and antihistamines. All prescription nasal sprays have the following common side effects:

a burning or itching sensation in the nose.

- Headache.
- Nausea.

These side effects can frequently be mitigated by altering your nasal spray technique. To avoid the spray's drip down your throat and subsequent motion sickness, tilt your head forward, for instance. Additionally, you may experience less pain if you direct the spray away from your nasal septum, which separates your left and right nostrils.

Decongestants

Decongestants can be taken orally or applied topically. Pseudoephedrine (Sudafed), one of the decongestants, can result in: when taken as a pill.

heart rate and blood pressure are both elevated.

Nervousness

urinary incontinence.

Decongestants can cause nasal dryness when used as a nasal spray, such as oxymetazoline (Afrin). Additionally, if you use a decongestant nasal spray for longer than three days in a row, your nose may grow accustomed to it, which could cause temporary worsening of the congestion when you stop using the medication. .

Ten Home Treatments for Seasonal Allergies

Your immune system overreacts to a particular trigger, such as weed, grass, or tree pollen, resulting in an allergy. As a result, the body produces antibodies and histamine, which arc then released into the bloodstream to combat the foreign substances. This sets off an inflammatory response that results in symptoms like itchy eyes, runny nose, congestion, sore throat, and sneezing.

Seasonal allergies in babies are possible

Allergies can affect anyone, but they typically begin after the age of three, peak in late childhood or the teen years, and then go away in adulthood. The onset of symptoms may occur in February and last through the end of September, depending on your location and the allergen. Antihistamines and steroid nasal sprays are two examples of medications that can offer relief, but there are also some natural DIY techniques that might be worth a try. The best home remedies for seasonal allergies are listed below for you to try.

Stay away from things that cause allergies

According to medical professionals, avoiding the allergens altogether is the best way to prevent symptoms in children who are prone to seasonal allergies. Keep abreast of the pollen counts in your area and take appropriate action. For instance, if you are aware that your child is allergic to ragweed, you should limit their time spent outside on days when the pollen count is at its highest. Although forcing kids inside during a beautiful day may seem cruel, experts say this tactic is actually very effective.

Prevent allergies in your home
Keep your windows closed, especially if the weather is warm and dry because that makes it simpler for pollen to fly through the air. At the beginning of the season, be sure to install a fresh filter in the air conditioning system, and replace it every two to three months. Use a dehumidifier

to reduce the humidity in your home because many allergens prefer moist environments. A portable high-efficiency particulate air (HEPA) filter is something else you might think about purchasing.

THE BEST ALLERGY DRUGS AND TREATMENTS FOR CHILDREN

The cling of pollen

Pollen sticks to skin, clothing, and almost anything else it touches, much like fine household dust. In the spring, you might see parked cars being dusted with a yellowish powder made of, for instance, oak pollen. Avoid hanging clothes, towels, or sheets outside to dry in order to keep it off your child. When your child enters the house, wipe their face, especially the area around their eyes, with a damp washcloth. Allowing your child to bathe or take a shower right before bedtime is recommended. If not, Robert Wood, M.D., warns that she will wake up all night reacting to the pollen in her head as she goes to sleep. , Baltimore's Johns Hopkins University Hospital's director of pediatric allergy clinics.

Keep your child's eyes safe

One of the most uncomfortable signs of allergies is teary, itchy eyes. The mucous membrane protecting the eye whites and inner eyelids becomes inflamed, which causes the itch. Keep pollen off your child's face to avoid the problem. Dr. Edith Schussler, M.D. , a pediatric allergist at

Weill Cornell Medicine in New York City, suggests putting on sunglasses and a brimmed hat. Kids frequently touch their faces, but if your child is wearing these accessories, they will be less likely to rub their eyes.

Use a saline solution as a last resort
Older kids may want to experiment with nasal irrigation using saline solutions, either purchased or made at home (most instructions call for combining distilled or boiled water with non-iodized salt). Clearing the nasal passages of mucus does just that. Neti pots can also be incredibly effective at clearing up congestion.

The correct way to use nasal spray.

Avoid smoking

Smoke from cigarettes should never be around any child who has known allergies because it may make their symptoms worse. Avoid going anywhere that has smoking in public.

Employ cold compresses

Try a cold compress, which can help lessen the itch and soreness, if your child has itchy eyes as a result of nasal allergies. Remind your children not to rub their eyes because doing so will only aggravate the itch and irritation.

Be sure to hydrate yourself

Yes, regular H_2O can do wonders. Because coughing and sneezing can dehydrate your child, it's crucial to consume enough fluids each day. Herbal teas, which have anti-inflammatory properties, are another option for your child to drink. Lastly, the steam from a hot bath or shower may help them to blow their stuffy nose.

Investigate potential substitute therapies

Alternative home remedies for seasonal allergies are incredibly popular among allergy sufferers. These include acupuncture, spirulina, stinging nettle, eucalyptus oil, and bromelain, an enzyme present in pineapple, as well as the plant known as butterbur (also known as Petasiteshybridus).

Eat foods that will lessen your allergies

The immune system can be strengthened and foods that produce naturally high quantities of vitamin C, zinc, vitamin D, antioxidants, and other beneficial vitamins and minerals are good options for preventing nasal allergies, according to ChitraDinakar, MdotD. at Children's Mercy Hospital in Kansas City, Missouri, who specializes in allergies.

Check out these choices.

Raspberry and blueberry fruits.

According to Jack Maypole, M.D., these contain vitamin C and flavanoids, which may lessen some of the histamine response for allergies in kids. , a pediatrician who serves on the educational advisory board of The Goddard School as well as an associate professor at Boston University School of Medicine. While conventionally grown versions of these fruits that have been well-washed are great and healthy additions, he notes that organic versions are always best. Elena Klimenko, M.D. , a New York City-based integrative medicine expert, concurs. Try consuming a serving of 3/4 cup once or twice per day, she advises. For young children who are still learning how to handle solids, thoroughly mash ripe berries.

Apples

In addition to flavanoids like quercetin, which can stabilize mast cells, these shiny orbs contain vitamin C. According to

Corinna Bowser, M.D, mast cells release histamine, making them significant mediators of allergy. a physician specializing in allergies at Narberth Allergy and Asthma in Narberth, Pennsylvania. When serving apples, it's best to peel and grate them because whole pieces of raw fruit pose a choking risk for children under the age of four. Alternatively, you could bake them until soft at 400 degrees F.

Onions: This vegetable also contains the antioxidant quercetin, though you might have a harder time convincing your child to eat onions. If so, this bulbous root, also known as allium cepa, can be eaten as pellets, according to Klimenko. Children over the age of two can use it safely if they follow the package instructions.

Honey

When it comes to reducing nasal allergies, this sweet treat gets mixed reviews, but it might be worth a try. According to Dr.dot Bowser, the theory behind it is that since pollen—which is the cause of allergies—is something that bees collect, eating honey regularly may help your body become accustomed to the allergen and prevent an allergic reaction. This theory has a flaw in that only wind-pollinated plants produce the pollen that causes allergic rhinitis, asthma, and allergic conjunctivitis, and honey contains only a small amount of pollen allergen, whereas allergens are primarily proteins. However, Dr. Klimenko suggests using local bee pollen. "Buy it seasonally and start with one to two granules, working up to a teaspoon a day," she advises. However, due to the risk of infant botulism, a serious gastrointestinal condition, honey should not be given to infants under the age of one.

spicier foods. Dishes made with cayenne pepper, fresh ginger, fenugreek, onions, and garlic may thin mucus and open nasal passages if your child is willing to try them. According to Dr.dot Bowser, the capsaicin present in spicy foods, such as red peppers, may work by desensitizing nasal nerve fibers.

When to Get Medical Attention for Allergies

Consult a doctor if your child's symptoms don't go away; the doctor may be able to identify allergies by looking over your child's medical history and conducting an examination. In some circumstances, the doctor may request some skin or blood tests to make a diagnosis.

Several allergy medications can safely and effectively reduce your child's symptoms. As an illustration, some antihistamines prevent the immune system from releasing histamine into the blood, preventing allergic reactions before they begin or slowing them down after they have started. Steroids, which are available as pills, eyedrops, nasal sprays, and oral liquids or liquids, work to reduce the inflammation brought on by the immune response. For some patients, allergy shots—the injection of very small amounts of an allergen—are beneficial; they work by triggering the production of antibodies against the allergen, preventing severe allergic reactions in the future.

Five Homeopathic Treatments for Seasonal Allergies

1. Your nasal passage should be cleaned.

Pollen adhering to your mucous membranes is one of the most frequent reasons for an allergy attack. If there is pollen present, your mucus membranes, or the glands lining the inside of your nose, will work extra hard to produce mucus. In order to lessen allergy symptoms, it's crucial to keep your nose clean.

The most popular method for clearing out your nasal passage and getting pollen off of your mucous membranes is using a neti pot. This nasal irrigation procedure resembles a tiny teapot that you fill with saline solution and pour through one nostril. Keep your head cocked so that the solution enters your other nostril. Even though it feels strange, you will feel much better after thoroughly rinsing your nasal passages with a neti pot. To keep pollen out of your nose and avoid allergy symptoms like sneezing and watery eyes, repeat this technique once or more throughout the day.

Even though they are extremely effective when used properly, a neti pot misuse could exacerbate symptoms and even lead to an infection. Here is an FDA-written manual on how to use a neti pot.

Aromatize essential oils

Using essential oils can be a great way to clear your nasal passages during allergy season. Any of your preferred essential oils will work, but those with menthol bases will be most effective at clearing your sinuses. Purified peppermint, spearmint, and eucalyptus oils should be purchased.

Smell them all day long.

Whatever method you choose, you'll soon be able to breathe easily and have your sinuses cleared up. You can simply twist the cap off the bottle and smell the oil, or you can purchase an essential oil diffuser so the room is filled with the scent, rub a few drops on your wrist, add some drops to your bath, or even add some to your tea.

Purge your house

Everybody who suffers from allergies should thoroughly clean their home. You probably bring allergy-triggering pollens inside from outside since seasonal allergies are linked to changes in the environment. In other words, even though you may feel like you're escaping the outside, they have probably entered your home to wreak havoc on your sinuses and adhere to your mucous membranes. Regardless of the specific plant to which you are allergic, there is a good chance that it has entered your house through open windows, carpeting, or clothing, or has been brought in on your shoes or clothing. Cleaning your home more frequently than usual will help you get through allergy season without going through ten boxes of tissues. You'll be grateful that you cleaned, vacuumed, and dusted everything.

Consider using herbal remedies

There are a few herbal treatments that have been reported to unclog sinuses and relieve allergy symptoms, but we'll only talk about quercetin and butterbur in this article. Quercetin is an antioxidant flavonoid that is present in a wide variety of plants and foods. As it works to stop the release of histamines, including this herb in your diet may help relieve common allergy symptoms. In a similar manner, butterbur functions as an antihistamine. Headaches, symptoms of seasonal allergies, and other conditions have all been known to be helped by this herb.

Take a Look at Acupuncture
Traditional Chinese medicine includes acupuncture, which has been shown to be effective in treating conditions like allergies and chronic pain. Although some people might not believe in this type of medicine, it is actually strongly supported by science. Discuss your allergy symptoms with an acupuncturist when you visit. Natural allergy relief with acupuncture includes relief from runny nose, itchy eyes, congested sinuses, and other symptoms.

An explanation of allergies
When a person reacts to environmental irritants that are normally safe for most people, they develop an allergy. As well as dust mites, pets, pollen, insects, ticks, mold, food, and some medications, these substances are also known as allergens.

The genetic propensity to develop allergic diseases is called atopy. Atopic individuals may experience an immune response that results in allergic inflammation when they are exposed to allergens. Those who experience this may exhibit the following symptoms.

- conjunctivitis and/or allergic rhinitis in the nose and/or eyes
- eczematous skin or skin hives (urticaria)
- asthma is caused by the lungs

What transpires in an allergic reaction?

An allergic reaction takes place when an allergen is in contact with a person who is allergic to it:

- An immune response is brought on when an allergen, such as pollen, enters the body

- Mast cells serve as a host for the antibodies

- Mast cells react by releasing histamine in response to the pollen coming into contact with the antibodies

- The inflammation (redness and swelling) that develops as a result of histamine release caused by an allergen is uncomfortable and upsetting

Some chemicals and food additives can cause comparable reactions. However, they are referred to as adverse reactions rather than allergies if the immune system is not involved.

What bodily regions could be impacted?

Depending on the allergen and how it enters the body, each person will experience a different set of symptoms. Multiple body parts may simultaneously be affected by allergic reactions.

- throat, sinuses, nose, and eyes.
- When an allergen is inhaled, histamine is released, causing the nasal lining to secrete more mucus and swell and inflame.
- It results in a runny, itchy nose and may make you sneeze ferociously.
- People might experience eye tearing up and a sore throat
- chest and the lungs
- Any allergic reaction has the potential to cause asthma. Breathing

becomes challenging when an allergen is inhaled because the lining of the airways in the lungs swells

- intestines and stomach
- Peanuts, seafood, dairy products, and eggs are among the foods that frequently cause allergies. Infants who are allergic to cow's milk may experience eczema, asthma, colic, and stomach discomfort
- Lactose, the milk sugar, is indigestible for some people.
- Stomach upsets are brought on by lactose intolerance, which is not the same as allergy
- Skin.

The skin conditions atopic dermatitis (eczema) and urticaria (hives) can be brought on by allergies.

Allergies that pose a life-threatening threat must be treated right away.

Most allergic reactions are mild to moderate and do not result in significant issues. Anaphylaxis, a severe allergic reaction that necessitates immediate life-saving medication, can happen to a small percentage of people. Food, insect, and medication allergies all have the potential to result in anaphylaxis. A severe allergy sufferer should have an ASCIA Action Plan for Anaphylaxis.

Options for treatment and prevention that work are available.

Finding the source of the allergy and taking action to lessen exposure to the allergen are necessary for allergen avoidance or minimization. People who are allergic to mites, for instance, may experience fewer symptoms if there are fewer dust mites in their home.

The following medicines are used to treat allergies:

Antihistamines prevent mast cell release of histamine, which lessens symptoms. Without a prescription, non-sedating antihistamine tablets can be purchased from pharmacies. Other options include the use of antihistamine nasal and eye sprays.

- When used correctly, intranasal corticosteroid nasal sprays (INCS) are effective for treating mild to severe allergic rhinitis.

- Stronger doses of INCS might need a prescription.

- Consult your physician or pharmacist for advice.

- In order to benefit from the benefits of both medications, combination therapies (INCS and antihistamine) are used to treat moderate to severe allergic rhinitis.

- Ask your doctor or pharmacist for advice if you think using medicated eye drops will help you.

Epinephrine, also known as adrenaline, is used to treat severe allergic reactions (anaphylaxis) that are life-threatening in an emergency situation. With an adrenaline autoinjector, which can be administered without medical training, adrenaline is typically administered.

Both allergic rhinitis and sinusitis can be treated without medication using saline sprays.

A long-term therapy called allergen immunotherapy, also referred to as desensitization, modifies how the immune system reacts to allergens. It entails giving regular, gradually increasing doses of allergen extracts via injections or sublingual tablets, sprays, or drops.

Herbal Treatments That Work to Beat Allergies

Narrow Leaf

Natural antihistamine nettle leaf can help to lessen swelling and relieve allergy symptoms. It can be consumed every day to help manage allergies and is available as a tea or supplement.

Quercetin

A flavonoid called quercetin can assist in stabilizing mast cells, which are in charge of releasing histamine during an allergic reaction. It is present in a wide variety of fruits and vegetables, such as apples, onions, and citrus fruits.

Butterbur

Natural treatment butterbur has been proven to be successful in easing allergy symptoms. Leukotrienes, which are chemicals that cause inflammation in the body, are blocked by this medication. The recommended dosage for butterbur, which is available as a supplement, is to be followed.

Honey produced nearby

By exposing your body to minute amounts of pollen, local honey is a natural remedy that can help lessen allergy symptoms. Since local honey will contain pollen from plants in your area, it is crucial to choose local honey.

We at Nao Medical are aware that dealing with allergies can be difficult. We provide a variety of services to assist you in managing your symptoms because of this. We're here to help you feel your best, offering everything from customized treatment plans to allergy testing.

13 home remedies for allergies that are natural and preventative

1. Examine nasal irrigation

According to OmidMehdizadeh, MD, an otolaryngologist (ENT) at Providence Saint John's Health Center, nasal irrigation with a saline rinse or spray is a fantastic first line of defense if someone is exhibiting nasal allergy symptoms, such as congestion or an itchy nose.

To loosen up the mucus and clear up congestion, you can first try purchasing a saline (saltwater) spray from your neighborhood grocery store and spritzing it in each nostril.

- Using a Neti Pot or another nasal irrigation tool is another option.

- You must adhere to the same instructions whether you're using a Neti Pot or a saline spray:.

- Tilt your head to the left, over the sink.

- Since the right nostril is the one that is highest, insert the tip of the instrument or spray bottle there.

- The remedy can be poured or sprayed in.

- Through the opposite nostril, the solution will exit.

- On the opposite side, repeat.

"The irrigations are the most effective because the patient is actually mechanically removing all the irritants from the nose. That might be useful in a lot of situations, says Mehdizadeh.

2. Acquire an air purifier

Your indoor allergies may improve if you buy a high-quality air purifier. Mehdizadeh claims that air purifiers, especially HEPA (high-efficiency particulate air) purifiers, are excellent at capturing indoor airborne allergens and lowering your risk of an allergic reaction.

Dust mites and pet dander are two typical indoor allergens that the purifier can help with.

3. Use a dehumidifier to prevent the growth of mold

Mehdizadeh advises reducing the humidity in your home if a mold allergy is more of a problem for you because mold grows and thrives in humid environments. Mehdizadeh recommends utilizing a dehumidifier in this situation.

Mehdizadeh advises using an adjustable dehumidifier at all times so you can manage how dry the space becomes. The nasal passages shouldn't become overly dry, as this can also be uncomfortable.

You can change the settings to reflect the EPA's recommendation that humidity levels be between 30 and 60 percent to prevent the growth of mold. Mehdizadeh advises against dipping below 30% because it can irritate the nose.

4. Diffuse the essential oils

Essential oils are strong, according to Mehdizadeh, so it's crucial to speak with your doctor before using them as an allergy treatment.

Having said that, some popular essential oils for allergies include:.

Lemon: The citrus essential oil of lemon is often used to treat allergies. By lowering inflammation and easing congestion, it functions as an antihistamine.

Natural menthol found in peppermint makes it an effective remedy for congestion and coughing. Inhaling menthol was found to relieve coughing more effectively than a placebo in a small 2013 study. This is accomplished by menthol's suppression of the cough reflex.

Eucalyptus: Eucalyptus oil has anti-inflammatory properties that help reduce airway inflammation and relieve nasal and chest congestion as a result.

Diffuser use is one method of utilizing these essential oils.

These essential oils are also available in dissolving shower tablets, so when the shower gets steamy, you can breathe in the aromas.

5. In the height of allergy season, wear a mask outside

Filtering out pollen and easing allergy symptoms can be accomplished with masks.

Wearing a face mask helped allergy sufferers avoid symptoms in their noses and eyes, according to a smaller study from 2021.

For the pollen count in your area, consult the weather. Wearing a mask outside may be advisable on days when there is a lot of pollen in the air.

6. Exclude allergens from your home

Make sure those outside allergens don't get inside your home if you suffer from seasonal allergies to plant pollen.

If you have an allergy to outdoor allergens, Mehdizadeh advises closing your windows.

More tips for protecting your home from pollen are provided below:

To keep allergens from circulating in your home's air, use a HEPA filter.

To prevent spreading allergens inside your home when you come inside from the outside, change into clean clothes and take a shower.

To prevent your pets from spreading allergens throughout your home, try to bathe them frequently.

7. Visit an acupuncturist on a scheduled appointment

Note: Only visit a licensed acupuncture professional. Finding a licensed acupuncturist in your area is as simple as conducting a search on the National Certification Commission for Acupuncture and Oriental Medicine's registry.

8. Consume a lot of vitamin C

Vitamin C, an antioxidant, can aid in the body's ability to combat inflammation and may even help with allergy symptoms.

The following are some sources of vitamin C.

- oranges, which are citrus fruits
- peppers—red and green
- Broccoli
- Bean sprouts
- Tomatoes

9. Don't smoke

Seasonal allergy symptoms may worsen if you are exposed to smoke, especially tobacco smoke. Even secondhand smoke can aggravate allergies and inflame the nasal passages.

Allergy sufferers may also be at risk from wildfire smoke, even in small amounts.

10.   Consider the spirulina

A microalga called spirulina is high in vitamins, minerals, and antioxidants. In addition to some grocery stores and pharmacies, it is available at health food stores.

Spirulina has a variety of health advantages, including a decrease in inflammation, in addition to providing relief from allergy symptoms.

11.   Exercise on a regular basis

Yoga could be a good alternative if you don't enjoy aerobic exercise. A small 2019 study involved eight weeks of three-times-weekly hatha yoga for a group of allergy sufferers. Due to decreased nasal blood flow and inflammation, patients who practiced yoga regularly experienced an improvement in their allergy symptoms.

Note: Check your local pollen count before planning to exercise outside during allergy season, and try to go when levels are lowest. alternatively, work out inside.

12.   Make sure you are getting enough vitamin D

The effectiveness of immunotherapy treatments may be improved by having adequate vitamin D levels in addition to reducing allergy symptoms. According to a small 2019 study, patients with adequate levels of vitamin D responded better to immunotherapy treatments.

The daily requirement for vitamin D in adults is 600 international units (IU).

It's crucial to note that consuming too much vitamin D can be harmful. Unless otherwise advised by a medical professional, don't take more than 4,000 IU per day.

13. Take local honey on a regular basis

By providing some exposure to pollen, local honey is thought to help lessen seasonal allergies.

Allergy Relief Through Natural Means.

As pollen from trees, grass, flowers, and plants enters the air, more than 35 million

Americans experience symptoms like sneezing, wheezing, runny noses, itchy, watery eyes, and redness.

Many people can find relief at the pharmacy counter thanks to the wide selection of conventional drugs that are available. Mother Nature, on the other hand, is the best road to relief for an increasing number of allergy sufferers, with a variety of all-natural treatments that studies show can help -- frequently without many of the unsettling side effects attributed to conventional treatment.

According to Mary Hardy, MD, director of integrative medicine at Cedars Sinai Medical Center in Los Angeles, "using nature-based products can be a very useful way to handle mild allergies and a useful adjunct for more significant allergies, and there are many types of treatments you can safely try."

Among those making the most noise at the moment is the European herb butterbur (Petasiteshybridus), which, according to Hardy, "has had some very impressive clinical trial results. ".

In a study that was recently published in the British Medical Journal, a team of Swiss researchers demonstrated how just one tablet of butterbur extract (Ze 339) taken four times per day was just as effective as a common antihistamine in reducing hay fever symptoms without causing the typical side effect of drowsiness. A second study that was presented at the 60th annual meeting of the American Academy of Allergy, Asthma, and Immunology (AAAAI) gave butterbur the thumbs-up for being effective in easing grass allergy symptoms.

According to Hardy, other herbal supplements that are working well include freeze-dried nettles and a tonic made from the herb goldenseal, which she suggests combining with one more all-natural remedy: a saline nasal spray (salt water).

Goldenseal has astringent and local antibacterial properties that can help in this process.

Many naturopathic doctors think that specific nutrients can be beneficial in reducing seasonal symptoms in addition to herbs. The most well-liked flavonoid substances are quercetin and grape seed extract. Although both are found in abundance in red wine and other foods, they can also be taken as supplements and have been shown to significantly lessen allergy symptoms, especially when combined with vitamin C.

You might want to consider preparing some hot, spicy foods to treat your allergies, shifting the focus from the medicine cabinet to the kitchen cabinet. The explanation: According to experts, hotter foods are more likely to thin mucous secretions, which can then clear nasal passages. Along with the conventional onion and garlic, the most frequently suggested spices for this use are cayenne pepper, hot ginger, and fenugreek.

Interestingly, your diet may not even be as important as your diet. Hardy hypothesizes that this is because seasonal allergies and food intolerance may be much more closely related than we realize.

Hardy advises cutting out any foods that even appear to cause mild sensitivity, such as sporadic hives or even stomach discomfort. She claims that by doing this, you can actually lessen the strain on your immune system, which in turn may help lessen the severity of seasonal allergic reactions.

From the Inside Out Seasonal Allergies

You might be tempted to try an air filtration system if your seasonal allergies are making you spend more time indoors than outdoors. According to many, these systems can remove bothersome dust and pollens from your personal space and thereby help with seasonal allergies. If this is the case, however, you should avoid doing so. But while these occasionally expensive units may clear the air, once an allergy is under way they don't seem to have much of an effect on symptoms, according to a recent report from the Agency for Health Care Research and Quality.

However, when outdoors in high pollen conditions, wearing a paper dust filter mask may work somewhat better.

You might experience a lot of relief by going to a doctor who practices the traditional Chinese medical technique known as acupuncture, in addition to any natural remedies you try on your own. In this case, treatment is thought to affect the immune system, where allergic reactions start, on the theory that stimulating points outside the body can change or initiate reactions inside.

Acupuncture reduced symptoms in all 26 participants in a small but significant study of 26 hay fever sufferers without any negative side effects, which was published in the American Journal of Chinese Medicine. In a second study, 72 participants, more than half of the participants had all of their symptoms completely resolved after just two treatments.

Due to its ability to calm immune system regions that have been overstimulated by exposure to numerous irritating factors, Dillard tells WebMD that acupuncture can be especially helpful if you have multiple allergies.

Although many alternative therapies can be very beneficial, allergist Marianne Frieri, MD, warns that natural doesn't always imply better or safer. She emphasizes that almost any substance found in nature's pharmacy has the potential to be toxic if used in excess and that it is possible to overdose on even the mildest-appearing medications.

She emphasizes the importance of never combining conventional medications with alternative therapies without your doctor's consent.

"For example, if you are taking the allergy drug Allegra, an antihistamine, at the same time you decide to try a natural substance with antihistaminic properties.

In addition, Hardy and Frieri warn against self-treating allergies if they are moderate to severe, even if you use natural remedies that seem safe. Always consult your allergist before doing so. Hardy claims that one key to success when attempting alternative medicine is beginning treatment before allergy symptoms appear. Three weeks before the start of allergy season is the ideal time to start, according to her.

Ginger is a low-cost, efficient alternative treatment for allergic rhinitis.

When the immune system overreacts to allergens in the air, allergic rhinitis, also known as hay fever, is a type of nasal inflammation. Runny or stuffy nose, sneezing, red, itchy, and watery eyes, and swelling around the eyes are some signs and symptoms. Typically, nasal discharge is clear.

The prevalence of allergic rhinitis is a serious global health issue. With 10 to 30% of adults and up to 40% of children experiencing it, it is the most prevalent type of non-infectious rhinitis. Epidemiological research shows that allergic rhinitis is becoming more common worldwide.

Antihistamines are among the most common medications used to treat allergic rhinitis. The goal of treatment has typically been to reduce these inflammatory reactions. Antihistamines, for example, can cause drowsiness, dry mouth, rash, and fatigue as side effects. For these reasons, it is imperative to look for a more tolerable substitute, particularly from herbs.

Everywhere in the world, ginger is used as a spice. It has been used as a component of herbal remedies in traditional Thai medicine to treat colds, constipation, insomnia, and flatulence. Ginger has been used in other medical systems, such as Indian and Chinese medicine, to treat a variety of ailments, including asthma, nausea, and arthritis.

Before the trial, they had given up taking antihistamines and intranasal steroids for a week, and they had no history of heart disease, kidney disease, liver disease, epilepsy, high blood pressure, or severe asthma.

The study's participants were told to follow the same course of treatment and take two capsules twice daily for six weeks; the experimental group received capsules containing ginger extract, while the control group received loratadine. Blood pressure monitoring, questionnaires, and blood analysis are used to gauge safety.

For the purpose of assessing the efficacy, safety, and patient compliance, all of them were followed up at the third and sixth week. Based on the study subjects' overall nose symptoms, such as runny nose, itchy nose, nasal congestion, and sneezing, the severity of allergic rhinitis was evaluated.

They claim that this research "showed that ginger extract could reduce allergic rhinitis symptoms and is safe to use with very mild gastrointestinal side effects like eructation. Ginger extract causes less drowsiness, fatigue, dizziness, and constipation than loratadine does.

Clinical trials have previously looked at ginger's efficacy in treating diseases like osteoarthritis, diabetes mellitus, motion sickness, nausea, and vomiting. There hasn't been any documented clinical evidence that ginger extract helps allergy sufferers with rhinitis, though.

How does Actifed Cold and Allergy work?

A mixture of chlorpheniramine and phenylephrine can be found in Actifed Cold and Allergy. An antihistamine, chlorpheniramine lowers the body's production of the histamine-related natural chemical. Runny nose, watery eyes, and sneezing are histamine-related symptoms. Decongestant phenylephrine constricts blood vessels in the nasal passages. Dilated blood vessels can cause nasal congestion (stuffy nose).

Sneezing, runny or stuffy nose, itchy, watery eyes, and other common cold and allergy symptoms are all treated with Actifed Cold and Allergy.

Warnings

Do not use Actifed cold and allergy medications if you have used MAO inhibitors such as isocarboxazid (Marplan), phenelzine (Nardil), rasagiline (Azilect), selegiline (Eldepryl, Emsam), or tranylcypromine (Parnate) in the past 14 days. Dangerous side effects may occur if you take Actifed Cold and Allergy before the MAO inhibitor has cleared from your body. Do not use this medication if you are allergic to chlorpheniramine or phenylephrine, or if you have severe high blood pressure or coronary artery disease, narrow-angle glaucoma, a stomach ulcer, or if you are unable to urinate.

In the event of an asthma attack, avoid using Actifed Cold and Allergy
Actifed Cold and allergy medications can cause side effects that slow thinking and reactions. Use caution when driving or doing anything that requires you to be awake and alert. Avoid drinking alcohol. It can increase some of the side effects of Actifed Cold and Allergy. The likelihood of this medication's side effects increasing with age. Always ask a doctor before giving cold medicine to a child. In very young children, misuse of cough and cold medications can result in death.

If symptoms do not improve or worsen after taking Actifed Cold & Allergy for 7 days, contact your physician.

Before taking this medicine

Do not use Actifed Cold and Allergy if you have used an MAO inhibitor such as isocarboxazid (Marplan), phenelzine (Nardil), rasagiline (Azilect), selegiline (Eldepryl, Emsam), or tranylcypromine (Parnate) within the past 14 days. Dangerous side effects may occur if you take Actifed Cold and Allergy before the MAO inhibitor has cleared from your body. Do not use Actifed Cold and Allergy if you are allergic to chlorpheniramine or phenylephrine, or if you have:.

- severe or uncontrolled high blood pressure
- severe coronary artery disease
- narrow angle glaucoma
- a stomach ulcer; or
- if you are unable to urinate

- Do not use Actifed Cold and Allergy tablets during an asthma attack

If you have certain conditions, you may need a dose adjustment or special tests to safely take this medication. Before you take Actifed Cold and Allergy, tell your doctor if you have:

- kidney disease
- liver disease
- diabetes
- glaucoma
- circulatory issues.
- high blood pressure or heart disease;.thyroid disease
- a seizure disorder, such as epilepsy
- or those who have chronic bronchitis, emphysema, or asthma

- issues with urination or a enlarged prostate

How is an overdose handled?

If you believe you have taken too much of this medication, seek emergency medical attention.

An overdose may result in stomach pain, nausea, vomiting, diarrhea, balance or coordination issues, headache, urination issues, dizziness, euphoria or irritability, hallucinations (seeing things), a metallic taste in your mouth, tremors, fever, flushed face, and seizures.

What ought I to stay away from?

Your thinking or behavior may be affected by the Actifed Cold and Allergy side effects.

When driving or performing other tasks that call for alertness and vigilance, use caution.

Try not to consume alcohol.

It may exacerbate some of Actifed Cold and Allergy's side effects.

Use of other sleep-inducing medications should be avoided (this includes muscle relaxants, cold medications, pain relievers, and medications for seizures, depression, or anxiety). They might intensify the drowsiness brought on by chlorpheniramine.

Refrain from taking additional medications (such as decongestants found in over-the-counter cold medications, caffeine, stimulants, diet pills, and others) that may make you restless. The stimulant effects of phenylephrine may be enhanced by them.

Effects of Actifed Cold and Allergy

If you experience any of the following symptoms after taking Actifed Cold and Allergy tablets: hives; difficulty breathing; swelling of your face, lips, tongue, or throat. If you experience any of these severe side effects from taking Actifed Cold and Allergy tablets, stop taking them immediately and call your doctor.

- heartbeats that are too quickly or irregularly

- feeling dizzy and passing out

- convulsions or seizures

- hallucinations (seeing things that aren't there); or

- tremors

The following list represents less severe side effects of Actifed Cold and Allergy.

- loss of appetite, nausea, vomiting, heartburn, and diarrhea

- mouth or nose are dry

- fatigue, vertigo, weakness, and headaches

- fuzzy vision and dry eyes

- Urination that is painful or challenging

- sleep issues (insomnia)

- (Especially in kids) feeling anxious or ecstatic.

Other side effects could occur; this is not a comprehensive list. For medical advice about side effects, contact your doctor. Call 1-800-FDA-1088 to report side effects to the FDA.

Actifed side effects (more information).

What other medications will affect Actifed Cold and Allergy?

Inform your doctor if you take any of the following medications before taking this medication:.

- Inversine's main ingredient is mecamylamine

- Aldomet, which contains methyldopa
- reserpine

Allergy to drugs.

The terms drug side effect and drug allergy are not interchangeable. A side effect is a recognized potential response to a medication. On their drug labels, medications list any potential side effects.

Drug toxicity differs from drug allergy.

An excessive dosage of medication results in drug toxicity.

Symptoms

After taking a medication, symptoms of a severe drug allergy frequently appear an hour later.

Hours, days, or even weeks later, there may be additional reactions, most notably rashes.

Symptoms of a drug allergy include:.

- Skin rashes
- Hives
- Itching
- Fever
- Swelling
- respiration difficulty
- Wheezing
- running nose
- watery eyes that itch

- Anaphylaxis

An uncommon, potentially fatal response to a drug allergy that results in widespread systemic dysfunction is known as anaphylaxis. Anaphylaxis symptoms include:

- breathing difficulty due to constriction of the throat and airways
- stomach pains or a nausea
- or diarrhea
- a feeling of faintness or dizziness
- swift and weak pulse
- lower blood pressure
- Seizure
- consciousness is lost
- Additionally afflicted by allergies to drugs

Less frequently, drug allergy reactions develop days or weeks after exposure to the drug and can last for some time after you stop taking it. Some of these circumstances are:

Serum sickness, which can result in fever, nausea, rash, swelling, and joint pain.

Drug-induced anemia, or a drop in red blood cells, can result in fatigue, erratic heartbeats, shortness of breath, and other symptoms.

Drug rash with eosinophilia and systemic symptoms (DRESS) causes a rash, high white blood cell count, general swelling, swollen lymph nodes, and recurrence of dormant hepatitis infection.

Nephritis, or kidney inflammation, can manifest as a fever, blood in the urine, generalized swelling, confusion, and other symptoms.

When to visit a doctor.

If you exhibit severe reaction symptoms or suspect anaphylaxis after taking a medication, call 911 or emergency medical assistance right away.

Consult your healthcare provider right away if you experience any drug allergy symptoms that are more subtle.

- Further details
- allergy to aspirin
- Schedule a meeting

Causes

A drug allergy happens when your body's immune system misinterprets a drug as a potentially dangerous substance, like a virus or bacteria. When a drug is identified by your immune system as being harmful, an antibody that is specific to that drug is created. Although an allergy may not manifest until after several exposures, this can occur when you take a drug for the first time.

These particular antibodies mark the drug and direct immune system attacks against it the following time you take it. This activity releases chemicals, which result in the symptoms of an allergic reaction.

However, you might be unaware of when you first used drugs.

According to some data, the immune system may be able to produce an antibody to a drug in the food supply in trace amounts, such as those found in antibiotics.

A slightly different process may be the cause of some allergic reactions. Some medications may be able to directly bind to the T cell, a specific type of immune system white blood cell. Chemicals that can cause an allergic reaction when you take the medication for the first time are released as a result of this event.

Drugs frequently associated with allergies

All medications have the potential to trigger an allergic reaction, but some medications are more frequently linked to allergies than others. These comprise:

- Penicillin is an antibiotic

- Aspirin, ibuprofen (Advil, Motrin IB, among others), and naproxen sodium (Aleve) are all examples of painkillers

- Cancer-treating drugs used in chemotherapy

- autoimmune disease medications, such as those for rheumatoid arthritis.

- drug reactions that are nonallergic

Symptoms of a drug reaction can occasionally resemble those of a drug allergy. However, immune system activity doesn't cause a drug reaction. The term "nonallergic hypersensitivity reaction" or "pseudoallergic drug reaction" refers to this condition.

The following medicines are more frequently linked to this condition:

- Aspirin.
- radiocontrast media (dyes) used in imaging tests.
- Opioids are used to treat pain.
- regional anesthetics.
- Added Details.
- Sulfa intolerance
- Risk elements

While anyone can experience an allergic reaction to a drug, certain things can make you more likely to do so.

These incorporate:

- a background of allergies, such as hay fever or food allergies

- a history of drug allergies in the family or personally

- exposure to a drug that has been increased due to high doses, frequent use, or prolonged use

- Certain diseases, like HIV infection or the Epstein-Barr virus, are frequently linked to allergic drug reactions

Prevention

The best defense against a drug allergy is to stop taking the offending substance. You can protect yourself by taking the following actions:

Inform the medical staff

In your medical records, make sure your drug allergy is clearly noted. Tell your dentist and any other medical specialists you may have about this.

www.ingramcontent.com/pod-product-compliance
Lightning Source LLC
Chambersburg PA
CBHW050816260726
48660CB00004B/1467